# Blood sugar revolution

**Blood Sugar Management: A Paradigm Shift in Diabetes Care**

By

# Morgan Williams

© 2023 by Morgan Williams
All rights reserved.

This publication is designed to provide general information regarding blood sugar management and diabetes care. It is not intended to replace medical advice or serve as a substitute for professional medical consultation. The publisher and author disclaim any liability arising directly or indirectly from the use of this material.

Cover design by Morgan Williams

# Table of contents

# Introduction

**The Blood Sugar Revolution signifies a transformative understanding of blood glucose management that has significant implications for health and well-being. This paradigm shift stems from a comprehensive comprehension of how blood sugar levels impact overall health,**

particularly in relation to conditions like diabetes.

Traditionally, blood sugar management primarily focused on monitoring and regulating glucose levels. However, the Blood Sugar Revolution encompasses a broader perspective. It involves not only recognizing the immediate effects of glucose imbalances but also understanding the intricate interplay between lifestyle, diet, genetics, and other factors that contribute to these fluctuations.

Central to this revolution is the realization that blood sugar levels are not solely influenced by sugary foods, but also by factors such as stress, sleep, physical activity, and gut health. This holistic understanding prompts individuals to adopt lifestyle changes that can have a profound impact on blood sugar stability and overall health.

Moreover, the Blood Sugar Revolution champions personalized approaches to blood glucose management. Thanks to advances in technology and medicine, individuals can now leverage wearable devices, continuous glucose monitors, and genetic insights to tailor interventions according to their unique physiological responses.

This revolution is marked by an emphasis on prevention rather than solely treatment. By proactively addressing blood sugar imbalances through dietary adjustments, regular exercise, stress reduction, and sleep optimization, individuals can reduce the risk of diabetes and other related health issues.

In essence, the Blood Sugar Revolution represents a shift from reactive management to proactive well-being. It encourages individuals to be more mindful of their daily choices, empowering them to take control of their health outcomes. Embracing this holistic understanding and adopting its principles can pave the way for a healthier and more balanced life, free from the shackles of blood sugar fluctuations and their associated health risks.

# Chapter 1

# What is blood sugar and its impact?

A crucial part of our body's energy management system is blood sugar, also referred to as blood glucose. It refers to the concentration of glucose, a type of sugar, present in the bloodstream. Glucose is the primary source of energy for our cells, especially the brain and muscles. Maintaining a balanced blood sugar level is crucial for overall health and well-being.

When we consume carbohydrates from foods like grains, fruits, and vegetables, our digestive system breaks them down into glucose, which then enters the bloodstream. The pancreas responds by releasing insulin, a hormone that helps cells absorb glucose from the blood to be used for energy or stored for later use.As a result of this procedure, blood sugar levels stay within the usual range.

However, disruptions in this balance can have significant impacts on health. If blood sugar levels become too high, a condition known as hyperglycemia occurs. This can happen in individuals with diabetes or those who consume excessive sugary or high-carbohydrate foods.

Chronic hyperglycemia can damage blood vessels, nerves, and organs over time, leading to complications such as heart disease, kidney damage, nerve problems, and vision impairment.

On the other hand, low blood sugar levels, or hypoglycemia, can result from skipping meals, excessive insulin or diabetes medication, or engaging in intense physical activity without proper fueling. Hypoglycemia can cause symptoms such as shakiness, confusion, dizziness, and even loss of consciousness. Severe cases can be life-threatening.

Maintaining a balanced blood sugar level is vital for everyone, not just individuals with diabetes. Consuming a balanced diet rich in whole grains, lean proteins, healthy fats, and fiber can help regulate blood sugar levels. Regular physical activity also plays a key role in glucose metabolism and insulin sensitivity.

Monitoring blood sugar levels, especially for those with diabetes, is essential. This can be done through regular blood tests and continuous glucose monitoring systems. Medications, lifestyle adjustments, and insulin therapy might be necessary to manage blood sugar effectively.

Blood sugar is a fundamental aspect of human physiology that impacts our energy levels and overall health. Striking a balance through a healthy diet, exercise, and proper medical

management is crucial to
prevent both short-term and
long-term complications
associated with high or low
blood sugar levels.

# Chapter 2

## The science of blood sugar

Blood sugar, also known as blood glucose, plays a critical role in the body's energy balance and overall health. It serves as the primary source of energy for cells and tissues, particularly the brain. The science of blood sugar regulation involves a complex interplay of hormones, organs, and cellular processes to maintain stable glucose levels.

The pancreas, a key player in
this process, releases insulin
and glucagon in response to
fluctuating blood sugar levels.
Insulin facilitates the uptake of
glucose from the bloodstream
into cells, particularly in
muscle and adipose tissue,
reducing blood sugar.
Meanwhile, glucagon raises
blood sugar levels by
promoting the release of stored
glucose from the liver.

The liver serves as a glucose
reservoir, releasing glucose
into the bloodstream between

meals or during periods of high demand. Muscle cells also store glucose as glycogen, which can be converted back into glucose when needed. This orchestrated dance of insulin, glucagon, and the liver's glycogen stores ensures a steady supply of glucose to maintain vital bodily functions.

When this delicate balance is disrupted, it can lead to health complications. Diabetes mellitus, a condition characterized by high blood sugar levels, is a result of insufficient insulin production or impaired cellular response to insulin. Chronic high blood sugar can damage blood vessels and nerves, contributing to cardiovascular disease, kidney damage, and neuropathy.

For controlling diabetes and minimizing complications, blood sugar monitoring is crucial.nAdvances in technology have led to the development of continuous glucose monitoring systems, providing real-time data for better control. Lifestyle modifications, such as a balanced diet, regular physical activity, and medications, are often prescribed to maintain healthy blood sugar levels.

The science of blood sugar regulation is a fascinating and intricate process involving multiple organs, hormones, and cellular mechanisms. Understanding this delicate balance and its implications for overall health is crucial for preventing and managing conditions like diabetes, ensuring optimal energy

utilization, and promoting
well-being.

**Factors influencing blood
sugar levels**

 Blood sugar levels are
influenced by a multitude of
factors that contribute to the
delicate balance of glucose in
the bloodstream. These factors
span from dietary choices and
physical activity to hormonal
interactions and overall health
status.

Diet is essential for controlling
blood sugar. Carbohydrates,

found in foods like grains, fruits, and vegetables, have the most direct impact. Simple carbohydrates can lead to rapid spikes in blood sugar, while complex carbohydrates provide a more gradual release. Fiber-rich foods can also help stabilize blood sugar by slowing down digestion and absorption.

Physical activity is another significant factor. Exercise increases glucose uptake by muscle cells, reducing blood sugar levels. Regular physical activity enhances insulin sensitivity, making cells more responsive to its effects, and thus promoting better blood sugar control.

Hormones, particularly insulin and glucagon, exert powerful influences on blood sugar levels. Insulin facilitates glucose uptake into cells, reducing blood sugar, while glucagon prompts the liver to release stored glucose, raising blood sugar. Hormonal imbalances, as seen in diabetes, disrupt this equilibrium.

Stress and emotional well-being impact blood sugar through hormonal responses. Stress hormones like cortisol can raise blood sugar levels, especially in individuals prone to insulin resistance. Sleep deprivation and chronic stress can contribute to elevated blood sugar levels over time.

Medications, especially for diabetes management, also affect blood sugar levels. Insulin injections, oral medications, and other treatments help regulate glucose by enhancing insulin

action or decreasing glucose
production.

Individual factors, such as
genetics and underlying health
conditions, influence blood
sugar levels. Genetic
predisposition can contribute
to a person's risk of developing
diabetes or experiencing
abnormal blood sugar
fluctuations. Other health
conditions, like hormonal
disorders or infections, can
temporarily impact blood
sugar control.

Blood sugar levels are intricately influenced by a range of factors, including diet, physical activity, hormones, stress, medications, genetics, and overall health. Understanding and managing these factors is crucial for maintaining stable blood sugar levels, preventing complications, and promoting overall well-being. Regular monitoring, healthy lifestyle choices, and appropriate medical interventions are key to achieving optimal blood sugar control.

# Types of Diabetes and their causes

Diabetes is a complex metabolic disorder characterized by
 blood sugar levels due to insufficient insulin production or poor utilization of insulin. There are three main types of diabetes: Type 1, Type 2, and gestational diabetes, each with distinct causes and underlying mechanisms.

**1. Type 1 Diabetes:** (Also known as insulin-dependent diabetes) Type 1 diabetes is an autoimmune condition where the body's immune system mistakenly attacks and destroys insulin-producing cells in the pancreas. As a result, little to no insulin is produced. Genetic predisposition and environmental factors, such as viral infections, are believed to trigger this immune response.

**2. Type 2 Diabetes:** The most common form, Type 2 diabetes, is characterized by insulin resistance, where cells do not respond effectively to insulin, and by inadequate insulin production over time. The onset of Type 2 diabetes is significantly influenced by lifestyle variables. Obesity, sedentary lifestyle, poor diet (high in sugary and processed foods), and genetics contribute to its onset. Age and ethnicity also play a role, with older adults and certain ethnic groups being more susceptible.

### 3.GestationalDiabetes:

Occurring during pregnancy, gestational diabetes is characterized by elevated blood sugar levels that develop in women who did not have diabetes before pregnancy. Hormonal changes during pregnancy can lead to insulin resistance, and some women's bodies may not be able to produce enough insulin to overcome it. Gestational diabetes typically resolves after childbirth, but it increases the risk of developing Type 2 diabetes later in life.

It's important to note that while these are the primary types of diabetes, there are also other, rarer forms, such as monogenic diabetes and secondary diabetes, which can result from specific genetic mutations or other underlying medical conditions.

Diabetes encompasses various types, each with its own causes and risk factors. Type 1 diabetes results from autoimmune destruction of insulin-producing cells, Type 2 diabetes is largely influenced by lifestyle and genetics, and gestational diabetes arises during pregnancy due to hormonal changes. Understanding these distinctions is essential for effective management and prevention strategies tailored to each type.

# Chapter 3

# Nutrition and blood sugar control

Nutrition plays a pivotal role in blood sugar control, with dietary choices directly influencing the body's ability to maintain stable glucose levels. A balanced and mindful approach to nutrition can help prevent and manage conditions like diabetes while promoting overall health.

Carbohydrates are a primary focus in blood sugar management. Choosing complex carbohydrates, such as whole grains, legumes, and vegetables, provides a slower release of glucose into the bloodstream, preventing rapid spikes. Monitoring portion sizes is also essential to prevent excessive carbohydrate intake.

Fiber-rich foods, including fruits, vegetables, whole grains, and nuts, are beneficial for blood sugar control. Fiber slows down digestion and absorption, causing blood sugar levels to rise more gradually. Additionally, fiber promotes satiety, aiding in

weight management and
overall glucose regulation.

Protein intake is important as
well. Including lean sources of
protein, such as poultry, fish,
tofu, and legumes, in meals
and snacks can help stabilize
blood sugar levels. Protein has
a minimal impact on blood
sugar and can contribute to a
feeling of fullness.

Healthy fats, like those found
in avocados, nuts, seeds, and
olive oil, are essential for
overall well-being and can
contribute to better blood

sugar control. They slow down the absorption of glucose, preventing rapid spikes, and support heart health.

Monitoring sugar intake is crucial. Limiting added sugars, sugary beverages, and processed sweets helps maintain stable blood sugar levels. Choosing whole fruits instead of fruit juices and opting for sugar-free or naturally sweetened options can reduce sugar consumption.

Meal timing and distribution also play a role. Regularly

eating balanced meals and snacks throughout the day helps lessen the likelihood of having drastic blood sugar swings. Skipping meals can lead to overeating later and disrupt blood sugar control.

Individualized meal planning and consulting a registered dietitian or healthcare professional are valuable steps for optimizing nutrition and blood sugar control. They can tailor recommendations to an individual's specific needs, taking into account factors like activity level, medication, and health goals.

Nutrition plays a vital role in blood sugar control. Emphasizing complex carbohydrates, fiber, lean proteins, healthy fats, and mindful portion control can help maintain stable glucose levels, prevent diabetes, and support overall well-being. A well-balanced and informed approach to eating is essential for promoting optimal health and blood sugar regulation.

# The role of carbohydrates, proteins, and fats on blood sugar

Carbohydrates, proteins, and fats are three macronutrients that play distinct and essential roles in the body, collectively contributing to overall health, energy production, and various physiological functions.

**Carbohydrates:** The body uses carbohydrates as its main source of energy. They are broken down into glucose, which fuels cells and tissues, particularly the brain and muscles. Complex carbs, which may be found in whole grains, veggies, and legumes, give you long-lasting energy since they take longer to digest and release glucose gradually. Simple carbohydrates, such as those in fruits and refined sugars, can lead to quick energy spikes. Fiber, a type of carbohydrate found in plant-based foods, supports digestion, helps maintain steady blood sugar levels, and promotes a feeling of fullness.

**Proteins:** Proteins are essential for building and repairing tissues, enzymes, hormones, and immune cells. They are made up of amino acids, which serve as the building blocks of the body. Proteins contribute to muscle development, tissue maintenance, and overall growth. Complete proteins, found in animal products like meat, fish, and dairy, contain all essential amino acids. Incomplete proteins, present in plant-based sources like beans, nuts, and grains, can be combined to create a complete amino acid profile. Protein also has a modest impact on blood sugar levels, making it a valuable nutrient for those managing diabetes.

**Fats:** Fats are integral to various bodily functions, including energy storage, hormone production, and cell structure. They offer a concentrated energy source and facilitate the assimilation of the fat-soluble vitamins (A, D, E, and K). Unsaturated fats, found in sources like avocados, nuts, and olive oil, support heart health by reducing LDL cholesterol levels. Omega-3 fatty acids, primarily found in fatty fish, have anti-inflammatory properties and contribute to brain health. Saturated fats, found in animal products and some plant oils, should be consumed in moderation, as excessive intake can increase LDL cholesterol and risk of cardiovascular disease.

Balancing these macronutrients is crucial for maintaining optimal health. A well-rounded diet should emphasize complex carbohydrates for sustained energy, lean proteins for tissue repair and growth, and healthy fats for essential functions. Individual dietary needs vary based on factors like age, activity level, and health conditions. Consulting a registered dietitian or healthcare professional can provide personalized guidance on macronutrient intake for overall well-being.

# Glycemic index and it's impact on blood sugar

The glycemic index (GI) is a numerical scale that measures how quickly and drastically a carbohydrate-containing food raises blood sugar levels when compared to a reference food, usually pure glucose or white bread. Understanding the GI of foods can be valuable for managing blood sugar levels, particularly for individuals with diabetes or those seeking to promote stable energy throughout the day.

High GI foods are quickly broken down, which causes a quick rise in blood sugar levels. Examples include sugary snacks, white bread, and white rice. These foods are quickly absorbed, leading to a surge in glucose in the bloodstream. This can be problematic for individuals with diabetes, as their bodies may struggle to regulate the sudden increase in blood sugar.

On the other hand, foods with a low GI are digested more

slowly, leading to a gradual
and more controlled rise in
blood sugar. Examples of
low-GI foods include whole
grains, legumes, most fruits,
and non-starchy vegetables.
These foods provide a more
sustained release of energy and
help prevent rapid fluctuations
in blood sugar levels.

The impact of the glycemic
index on blood sugar is not the
sole consideration for healthy
eating. Portion size, nutrient
composition, and the presence
of fiber and fat also influence
how a food affects blood sugar.

Combining foods with varying GI values can also impact overall blood sugar response. For example, consuming a high-GI food along with protein or healthy fats can help moderate the rise in blood sugar.

Managing the glycemic index of foods can be particularly beneficial for individuals with diabetes. Monitoring and choosing low to moderate-GI foods can aid in better blood sugar control and reduce the risk of hyperglycemia (high blood sugar) or hypoglycemia (low blood sugar) episodes. However, it's important to note that the GI is just one tool among many for making healthy food choices. A well-balanced diet that includes a variety of nutrient-dense foods is key for overall health and blood sugar management.

The glycemic index is a valuable concept that helps individuals make informed dietary choices to manage blood sugar levels. Low to moderate-GI foods provide a more gradual release of

glucose, promoting stable
energy and supporting overall
health, especially for those
with diabetes.

# Designing a blood sugar-friendly diet plan

Designing a blood
sugar-friendly diet plan
involves thoughtful
consideration of the types and
timing of foods to help
maintain stable glucose levels.

This approach is especially important for individuals with diabetes, as well as those aiming to prevent blood sugar fluctuations and promote overall well-being.

## 1. Emphasize Complex Carbohydrates:

Choose whole, unprocessed carbohydrates with a low to moderate glycemic index (GI). Opt for whole grains like quinoa, brown rice, and whole wheat over refined options. Incorporate a variety of fruits and non-starchy vegetables, as they provide fiber and

nutrients while having a
milder impact on blood sugar.

## 2. Include Lean Proteins:
Incorporate lean sources of
protein such as poultry, fish,
tofu, legumes, and low-fat
dairy. Protein helps stabilize
blood sugar levels and
promotes satiety, reducing the
risk of overeating or snacking
on high-sugar foods.

## 3. Healthy Fats: Select
heart-healthy fats like
avocados, nuts, seeds, and
olive oil. These fats slow down

digestion, preventing rapid spikes in blood sugar. Include fatty fish rich in omega-3 fatty acids, as they offer anti-inflammatory benefits.

## 4. Portion Control: Pay attention to portion sizes to avoid overeating. Eating smaller, balanced meals and snacks throughout the day can help prevent large swings in blood sugar levels.

## 5. Fiber-Rich Foods: Prioritize fiber-rich foods like whole grains, vegetables, and legumes. Fiber helps control

blood sugar levels and slows down digestion.

## 6. Limit Added Sugars and Refined Carbs:

**Minimize consumption of sugary foods, sugary beverages, and refined carbohydrates. These may cause sharp rises in blood sugar.**

## 7.Balanced Meals and Snacks:

**Aim for balanced combinations of carbohydrates, proteins, and fats in each meal and snack.**

This lessens the chance of blood sugar spikes.

## 8. Regular Eating Schedule: Establish a consistent eating schedule to regulate blood sugar levels. Skipping meals can lead to overeating later and disrupt glucose balance.

## 9. Drink plenty of water all day long to stay hydrated: Proper hydration supports overall health and can help control appetite and blood sugar levels.

## 10. Consult a Professional:

Work with a registered dietitian or healthcare provider to create a personalized blood sugar-friendly diet plan. They can consider individual preferences, health goals, and any medical conditions to tailor recommendations.

Creating a blood sugar-friendly diet plan involves a holistic approach that incorporates a variety of nutrient-dense foods, mindful eating practices, and regular monitoring. A well-designed plan can contribute to stable blood sugar levels, reduce the risk of complications, and promote optimal health.

# Chapter 4

# Lifestyle strategies for optimal blood sugar

Optimal blood sugar control is crucial for overall health, particularly for individuals with diabetes or those seeking to prevent blood sugar imbalances. A combination of lifestyle strategies can significantly contribute to achieving and maintaining stable blood sugar levels.

## 1. Regular Physical Activity: Engaging in regular exercise helps improve insulin

sensitivity, allowing cells to more effectively use glucose for energy. Aim for a mix of aerobic and strength-training exercises, and consult a healthcare provider before starting a new exercise routine.

## 2. Healthy Eating Habits:

Prioritize whole, nutrient-dense foods. Choose lean proteins, complex carbs, and healthy fats. Control portion sizes to prevent overeating and monitor carbohydrate intake to manage blood sugar levels.

### 3. Balanced Meals and Snacks: Plan well-balanced meals and snacks that include a combination of carbohydrates, proteins, and fats. This combination helps stabilize blood sugar levels and prevents rapid spikes.

### 4. Regular Meal Timing: Establish consistent meal and snack times to regulate blood sugar levels. Avoid skipping meals, as it can lead to overeating later and disrupt glucose balance.

**5. Maintaining proper hydration throughout the day by consuming water.** Proper hydration supports overall well-being and can help control appetite and blood sugar levels.

**6. Stress Management:** Chronic stress can impact blood sugar levels. Incorporate stress-reduction techniques such as meditation, deep breathing, yoga, or engaging in hobbies.

**7. Adequate Sleep:**
Prioritize getting enough quality sleep each night. Sleep deprivation can affect insulin sensitivity and lead to blood sugar imbalances.

**8. Limit Alcohol Consumption:** If you choose to consume alcohol, do so in moderation and be mindful of its impact on blood sugar. Alcohol can lead to fluctuations and should be consumed along with food.

**9. Regular Monitoring:**
For individuals with diabetes,

consistent blood sugar monitoring is essential. This helps identify patterns and make necessary adjustments to medication or dietary habits.

## 10. Consult Healthcare Professionals: Work with a healthcare team, including a registered dietitian and physician, to create a personalized plan tailored to your specific needs, health goals, and medical conditions.

## 11. Weight Management: Achieving and maintaining a healthy weight can improve

insulin sensitivity and blood sugar control. A balanced diet and regular exercise play key roles in weight management. Adopting these lifestyle strategies can contribute to optimal blood sugar control and support overall well-being. Consistency and ongoing monitoring are essential for successful blood sugar management, especially for individuals with diabetes. Making gradual, sustainable changes to your lifestyle can lead to lasting improvements in blood sugar levels and overall health.

# Exercise and physical activity guidelines

Exercise and physical activity are integral components of a healthy lifestyle, offering a wide range of benefits for both physical and mental well-being. Following established guidelines can help individuals of all ages and fitness levels reap the rewards of regular physical activity.

## 1:Aerobic Exercise:

Aerobic activities, also known as cardiovascular exercise, elevate heart rate and breathing. Aim for 75 minutes of strong aerobic exercise or 150 minutes of moderate aerobic exercise per week. Activities can include brisk walking, jogging, swimming, cycling, dancing, or playing sports.

## 2:Strength Training:

Incorporating strength training exercises at least two days a week helps build and maintain muscle mass. Focus on all major muscle groups, such as legs, arms, back, chest, and core. Free weights, resistance bands, or body weight exercises like push-ups and squats are effective options.

## 3:Flexibility and Stretching: Engage in flexibility exercises to improve joint range of motion and prevent injury. Incorporate stretching exercises that target major muscle groups and hold each stretch for 15-30 seconds. Yoga and Pilates are excellent

choices for enhancing
flexibility.

## 4:Balance Training:

Especially important for older
adults, balance exercises help
prevent falls and improve
stability. Simple activities like
standing on one leg or Tai Chi
can enhance balance and
coordination.

# Guidelines for All Ages:

**-Children and Adolescents (6-17 years):** Aim for at least 60 minutes of moderate-to-vigorous physical activity daily, including a mix of aerobic, strength, and bone-strengthening activities.

**- Adults (18-64 years):** Aim for 150-300 minutes of moderate-intensity aerobic exercise per week, along with muscle-strengthening activities on two or more days.

**- Older Adults (65+ years):** Follow the adult guidelines if possible, focusing on activities that enhance balance and flexibility. Consult a healthcare provider for guidance if needed.

# Additional Considerations

**- Gradual Progression:**
Start slowly if you're new to exercise and gradually increase intensity and duration to prevent injury.

**- Observe Your Body:** Pay attention to how your body feels after working out.. Adjust intensity or rest as needed.

**- Variety:** Incorporate a mix of aerobic, strength, flexibility, and balance activities to promote overall fitness.

- **Warm-Up and Cool-Down:** Begin each session with a 5-10 minute warm-up and end with a 5-10 minute cool-down to prepare the body and aid recovery.

Remember, any amount of physical activity is beneficial. Before beginning a new workout regimen, especially if you have any underlying medical concerns, speak with a healthcare professional. By following these exercise and physical activity guidelines, you can enjoy improved health, enhanced fitness, and a higher quality of life.

# Stress management and it's influence on blood sugar

Stress management plays a pivotal role in maintaining overall well-being, particularly in its profound impact on blood sugar levels. In today's fast-paced world, chronic stress has become a prevalent issue, often leading to a range of health concerns, including diabetes and blood sugar fluctuations.

When the body experiences stress, it triggers the release of stress hormones such as cortisol and adrenaline. These hormones prepare the body for the "fight or flight" response by increasing heart rate, redirecting blood flow, and releasing glucose into the bloodstream. This surge in glucose is meant to provide quick energy for physical exertion. However, in the context of chronic stress, the frequent release of these stress hormones can disrupt the body's delicate balance.

One significant connection between stress management and blood sugar lies in the increased risk of developing type 2 diabetes. Prolonged stress can lead to insulin resistance, where cells become less responsive to insulin, the hormone that regulates blood sugar. This resistance can result in elevated blood sugar levels, increasing the likelihood of diabetes over time.

Effective stress management techniques play a crucial role in mitigating these effects. Regular physical activity, mindfulness practices like meditation and deep breathing, and maintaining a balanced diet are all essential components of stress management. Engaging in these activities helps lower stress hormone levels, promote insulin sensitivity, and stabilize blood sugar levels.

Moreover, a positive feedback loop exists between stress and blood sugar: elevated blood sugar levels due to stress can, in turn, contribute to more stress and exacerbate the cycle. By managing stress, individuals can break this cycle and prevent the further deterioration of their blood sugar regulation.

Stress management is a cornerstone of maintaining optimal health, and its impact on blood sugar levels cannot be underestimated. Chronic stress can lead to insulin resistance and higher blood sugar levels, increasing the risk of diabetes and related complications. Prioritizing stress reduction through various methods can positively influence blood sugar regulation, helping to prevent the onset of diabetes and promoting overall well-being.

# Chapter 5

## Natural and integrative therapies

Natural and integrative therapies encompass a diverse array of holistic approaches that focus on enhancing health and well-being through a combination of conventional and complementary practices.

Embracing the principles of treating the whole person—mind, body, and spirit—these therapies aim to address underlying causes rather than merely alleviating symptoms.

At the core of natural and integrative therapies is the belief in the body's innate ability to heal itself. This approach emphasizes the use of natural remedies, lifestyle modifications, and alternative therapies to promote healing and prevent illness. From herbal medicine and acupuncture to chiropractic care and nutritional counseling, these therapies draw from both ancient traditions and modern research.

One of the central tenets of integrative therapies is the importance of individualized treatment. Practitioners work closely with patients to create personalized plans that consider their unique medical history, current health status, and goals. By fostering a collaborative and patient-centered approach,

integrative therapies empower
individuals to take an active
role in their health journey.

A hallmark of natural and
integrative therapies is their
emphasis on prevention.
Rather than waiting for health
issues to arise, these therapies
focus on optimizing health and
well-being to prevent illness
from occurring in the first
place. This proactive approach
often includes promoting a
balanced diet, regular exercise,
stress reduction techniques,
and adequate sleep.

While integrative therapies are often used as complementary approaches alongside conventional medical treatments, they can also play a central role in managing chronic conditions. Conditions such as chronic pain, anxiety, and autoimmune disorders have been shown to respond positively to a combination of conventional and natural therapies.

It's important to note that natural and integrative therapies are not a one-size-fits-all solution, and their effectiveness may vary from person to person. Consulting qualified healthcare professionals and practitioners is essential to ensure safe and appropriate use of these therapies, especially when integrating them with conventional medical treatments.

 Natural and integrative therapies offer a holistic approach to health and healing that considers the interconnectedness of the mind, body, and spirit. By combining ancient wisdom

with modern science, these
therapies empower individuals
to take charge of their
well-being and promote a
balanced, proactive approach
to health that goes beyond
symptom management.

# Herbal remedies and supplements

Herbal remedies and
supplements have a long
history as natural alternatives

to conventional medicine, offering a diverse range of potential health benefits. Derived from plant sources, these remedies have been used for centuries in various cultures to address a wide array of health concerns. While they can provide valuable support, it's essential to approach their use with caution, understanding their potential benefits and risks.

Herbal remedies encompass a wide variety of plant-based substances, including leaves, roots, flowers, and seeds.

These natural compounds contain bioactive components that can have therapeutic effects on the body. For instance, herbs like echinacea are believed to boost the immune system, while valerian root is often used for its potential to promote relaxation and sleep.

Supplements, on the other hand, include vitamins, minerals, and other dietary compounds that are often consumed in concentrated forms to augment one's nutritional intake. Common examples include vitamin D, omega-3 fatty acids, and probiotics. Supplements are commonly used to address specific deficiencies or enhance overall well-being.

While herbal remedies and supplements can offer benefits, it's important to note that their efficacy can vary widely. Scientific research on their effects is still evolving, and regulatory oversight may be less stringent than that for conventional medications. Consultation with a healthcare professional is crucial before

introducing any herbal
remedy or supplement into
your routine, especially if you
have pre-existing health
conditions, are taking other
medications, or are pregnant
or breastfeeding.

Another aspect to consider is
potential interactions. Some
herbal remedies and
supplements can interact with
prescription medications,
potentially affecting their
effectiveness or causing
adverse effects. A healthcare
provider can help you navigate
these complexities and make

informed decisions about incorporating these products into your health regimen.

 Herbal remedies and supplements offer a natural approach to health and well-being, drawing on the potential therapeutic properties of plant-based compounds and concentrated nutrients. While they can be beneficial, it's important to approach their use with caution, seeking guidance from healthcare professionals and being mindful of potential interactions or side effects. An

informed and balanced
approach can help you harness
the potential benefits of these
natural remedies while
prioritizing your overall health
and safety.

# Acupuncture, Yoga, and Mind-Body practice

Acupuncture, yoga, and
mind-body practices are
powerful and time-tested
methods that contribute to

holistic well-being, fostering a harmonious connection between the mind, body, and spirit. These practices have garnered increasing attention for their potential to enhance physical health, reduce stress, and promote mental clarity.

**Acupuncture**, an ancient Chinese therapy, involves the insertion of thin needles into specific points on the body's energy pathways, known as meridians. This practice aims to balance the flow of energy, or  stimulate the body's natural healing mechanisms.

Acupuncture has been linked
to pain relief, stress reduction,
and improved energy flow.

**Yoga**, originating in ancient
India, encompasses a range of
physical postures, breathing
techniques, and meditation
practices. It promotes
flexibility, strength, and
relaxation, while also fostering
mindfulness and
self-awareness. Regular yoga
practice has been associated
with reduced stress, improved
posture, and enhanced mental
focus.

**Mind-body practices** encompass a broad spectrum of techniques, including meditation, deep breathing, and guided imagery. These practices emphasize the profound connection between mental and physical health. Mindfulness meditation, for example, encourages being present in the moment, reducing anxiety and promoting emotional well-being. Deep breathing techniques can activate the body's relaxation response, leading to reduced stress and a sense of calm.

Collectively, these practices offer numerous benefits for individuals seeking to achieve balance and vitality in their lives. They can help manage chronic pain, reduce anxiety and depression, enhance sleep quality, and promote overall resilience. Furthermore, the integration of these practices into healthcare settings is becoming more common as their therapeutic potential gains recognition.

While these practices hold promise, it's important to note

that their effects can vary from person to person. They are often best utilized as complementary approaches alongside conventional medical care. Consulting with qualified practitioners and healthcare professionals can help tailor these practices to individual needs and health conditions.

Acupuncture, yoga, and mind-body practices provide valuable tools for cultivating well-being on multiple levels. They empower individuals to tap into their body's innate healing abilities, fostering physical health, mental clarity, and emotional balance. By integrating these practices into one's lifestyle and seeking guidance when needed, individuals can embark on a journey toward holistic wellness and self-discovery.

# Integrating complementary approaches with medical treatment

Integrating complementary approaches with medical treatment is a progressive and holistic approach that recognizes the potential benefits of combining conventional medical care with complementary therapies. This synergistic approach aims to provide comprehensive and well-rounded healthcare, addressing not only the physical symptoms but also considering the individual's emotional, mental, and spiritual well-being.

Complementary approaches encompass a diverse range of practices, including acupuncture, herbal medicine, yoga, meditation, and massage therapy, among others. These therapies are often used in conjunction with conventional medical treatments to enhance their effectiveness, alleviate side effects, and promote overall well-being.

One significant advantage of integrating complementary approaches is the potential to provide a more personalized and patient-centered care experience. These therapies can be tailored to the individual's unique needs and preferences, fostering a deeper connection between the patient and their healthcare providers.

Moreover, complementary approaches can fill gaps where conventional treatments may fall short. For instance, acupuncture and mindfulness techniques have shown promise in managing chronic pain and reducing stress, supplementing pain medications and enhancing overall pain management strategies.

Integrating complementary approaches also acknowledges the interconnectedness of the mind and body. Emotional and psychological well-being play a crucial role in physical health, and practices such as meditation and relaxation techniques can contribute to reduced anxiety, improved mood, and better treatment outcomes.

However, it's essential to approach this integration with

care and open communication. Healthcare professionals should be involved in the decision-making process to ensure that complementary therapies are safe, appropriate, and compatible with the individual's medical condition and treatment plan.

Integrating complementary approaches with medical treatment offers a comprehensive and patient-centered approach to healthcare. By harnessing the potential benefits of both conventional medicine and complementary therapies, individuals can experience a more holistic and well-rounded approach to healing. This approach recognizes the diverse needs of patients and seeks to optimize their overall well-being by considering all aspects of their health journey.

# Chapter 6

## Personalizing blood sugar management

**Personalizing blood sugar management is a crucial and**

evolving approach that recognizes the unique physiological and lifestyle factors that impact an individual's blood sugar levels. It involves tailoring diabetes management strategies to each person's specific needs, preferences, and circumstances, with the goal of achieving optimal blood sugar control and overall well-being.

Every individual's response to food, exercise, medication, stress, and other factors can vary significantly. Personalizing blood sugar management involves closely monitoring these variables and adjusting treatment plans accordingly. Continuous glucose monitoring (CGM) technology, for example, provides real-time data on blood sugar levels, enabling individuals and healthcare providers to make informed decisions in real-time.

Diet plays a pivotal role in blood sugar management, and personalization extends to creating individualized meal plans. Considering factors such as carbohydrate intake, glycemic index, and timing of meals can help stabilize blood sugar levels. Some individuals might respond well to a low-carbohydrate diet, while others may find success with a balanced approach.

Physical activity is another crucial component, with personalized exercise routines designed to help regulate blood sugar levels. Tailoring exercise plans to an individual's fitness level, preferences, and glucose response can optimize the benefits of physical activity.

Medication management is also personalized, taking into account an individual's medication sensitivities and potential interactions. For those with type 2 diabetes, various oral medications and insulin regimens can be tailored to achieve target blood sugar levels while minimizing side effects.

Stress and emotional well-being are often overlooked but play a significant role in blood sugar management. Techniques such as mindfulness, meditation, and stress reduction strategies can be personalized to address emotional triggers that affect blood sugar levels.

Collaboration between healthcare providers and individuals is essential in personalizing blood sugar management. Regular check-ins, data sharing, and open communication help fine-tune treatment plans over time.

 Personalizing blood sugar management is a dynamic and comprehensive approach that recognizes the unique factors influencing blood sugar levels. By tailoring diet, exercise, medication, stress management, and other aspects of diabetes care to individual needs, individuals can achieve better blood sugar control and ultimately improve their quality of life. This personalized approach acknowledges that managing diabetes is not a one-size-fits-all endeavor and empowers individuals to take an active role in their health journey

# Genetics and Individual variability

Genetics and individual variability are intertwined factors that contribute to the unique characteristics and responses of each person. Human genetics play a significant role in shaping various aspects of an individual's health, physical traits, and susceptibility to diseases. However, it is the intricate interplay between genetics and environmental influences that leads to the remarkable diversity observed among individuals.

Genetics forms the foundation of an individual's inherited traits, determining factors such as eye color, height, and predisposition to certain health conditions. The Human Genome Project has deepened our understanding of genetic makeup, revealing insights into how specific genes influence various aspects of health and disease.

Yet, individual variability goes beyond genetics. Environmental factors, lifestyle choices, and experiences also play a crucial role in shaping an individual's health outcomes. Nutrition, exercise, stress levels, and exposure to toxins are just a few examples of external influences that interact with genetic predispositions.

The field of personalized medicine capitalizes on the concept of individual variability. By analyzing an individual's genetic makeup and considering their unique lifestyle and environmental factors, healthcare providers can tailor treatment plans to optimize effectiveness and minimize adverse effects. This approach is particularly relevant in areas like cancer treatment, where specific genetic mutations can influence how a person responds to therapies.

Understanding individual variability also highlights the importance of a patient-centered approach in healthcare. Recognizing that

each person is unique helps
healthcare professionals
develop treatment strategies
that align with the patient's
preferences, values, and
circumstances.

Moreover, the study of genetics
and individual variability has
implications beyond
healthcare. It has a significant
impact on fields such as
education, psychology, and
even social sciences. Research
into the genetic basis of
learning styles or personality
traits, for instance, contributes

to a deeper understanding of human diversity.

Genetics and individual variability are intertwined factors that contribute to the rich tapestry of human life. While genetics lay the groundwork for inherited traits, individual variability emerges from the complex interplay between genes, environment, and lifestyle. Recognizing and embracing this diversity not only advances scientific knowledge but also informs personalized

approaches to healthcare,
education, and beyond.

# Conclusion

The concept of the "Blood
Sugar Revolution"
underscores the
transformative journey
towards a more personalized
and holistic approach to blood
sugar management. This
revolution encompasses a shift
from traditional,

one-size-fits-all strategies to tailored interventions that consider an individual's unique physiological, genetic, and lifestyle factors.

The revolution in blood sugar management has highlighted the critical role of personalized care. By recognizing that no two individuals are alike, healthcare professionals are better equipped to develop targeted treatment plans that optimize blood sugar control and overall well-being. This individualized approach takes into account factors such as genetics, dietary preferences, exercise habits, stress levels, and medication sensitivities, resulting in more effective and sustainable outcomes.

Furthermore, the Blood Sugar Revolution emphasizes the integration of complementary approaches with conventional medical care. Practices like acupuncture, yoga, and mindfulness techniques have demonstrated their potential to complement standard treatments, enhancing blood sugar regulation and promoting emotional resilience.

Continuous glucose monitoring (CGM) technology has also played a pivotal role in this revolution, providing real-time data that empowers individuals to make informed decisions about their daily activities, food choices, and medication management. The availability of such data fosters a sense of empowerment and ownership over one's health, leading to better self-management and treatment adherence.

The Blood Sugar Revolution represents a paradigm shift in the management of blood sugar levels. It embraces the diversity of individuals and acknowledges the intricate interplay between genetics, lifestyle, and environment. By tailoring interventions, embracing complementary practices, and leveraging advanced technologies, this revolution paves the way for a future where blood sugar management is not only more effective but also more personalized and empowering.

As healthcare continues to evolve, the principles of the Blood Sugar Revolution serve as a beacon of hope, guiding us towards a more holistic and individual-centric approach to improving the lives of those affected by blood sugar imbalances.

# TNTRIO MOVEMENT

## BOOK - 5

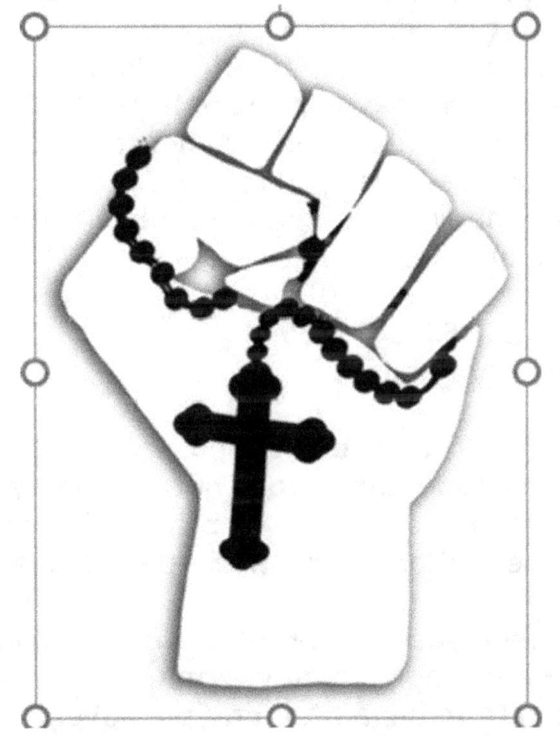

### Franklin Ysaac + Eliseo Rio Jr. + Gus Guzman

April 2023

Published in USA in May 2023 by
TATAY JOBO ELIZES,
Self-Publisher, under the permission and
authorization of

# Franklin Ysaac, et al
authors and copyright owners.



KDP ISBN: *9798393478865*
Independently Published



Contact: job_elizes@yahoo.com +
https://www.facebook.com/franklin.ysaac +
http://tinyurl.com/mj76ccq (amazon site) +
www.tatayjoboelizes.webs.com +
https://www.facebook.com/groups/399368500835109